Melody's Battle

By Mary Kristofek

This book is dedicated to all people who suffer from Alzheimer's disease or dementia, and their caregivers.

CONTENTS

ACKNOWLEDGMENTS

A very special thanks to Beth, Joyce and Tammy. Without their help and guidance during Melody's battle, I know I wouldn't have made it through the long and difficult years.

I'm very grateful to my mother, Barbara. When we talked on the phone daily, she always knew from the tone of my voice the times that Melody and I were having a challenging day. She wasn't able to be there physically but was always there for moral support, especially the times when I needed a good cry.

Thank you to the professionals at Total Longterm Care Center, Ashley Manor Assisted Living and Bethany Nursing Home Hospice.

Finally, I'd like to thank my partner of three years, Stacie, who inspired me to journal and write this book. Her countless hours spent editing and typing made this book possible.

Chapter 1

Melody and Mary's Family History

Melody was born in Flint, Michigan in 1952. She had one older sibling, Dawn, who was born in 1949. Dawn passed away on January 2nd, 1999, from bladder cancer. She was only 49 years old. The two were very close, and Melody traveled back and forth from Colorado to Michigan during Dawn's fight with cancer. Melody was by Dawn's side when she died.

Melody went through a lot of depression and guilt after her sister died. She felt like her life should have been taken instead of Dawn's, because she herself had no children, and Dawn was a single mom with two daughters. Dawn's two daughters, Angie and Kristy, continued to have a relationship with Melody after Dawn's death. Melody had a half-brother, Joel, who lives in Michigan, and a half-sister, Beverly, who lives in Florida. Melody was always close to Joel, and they talked regularly on the phone during her early stages of dementia.

Melody and Dawn's parents are deceased. Her father Elmer died from bladder cancer in his mid 60's, and her mother Ellen passed away from Alzheimer's disease, at the age of 78. Ellen suffered from mental illness, and did some bizarre things when Melody was little. Melody was a Halloween baby, and every year Ellen would show up at Melody's grade school, dressed like a scary witch. One year she scared many of the children, so they banned her from ever coming to the school dressed up again.

I was born in Arizona on September 11th, 1960. I have four siblings, Tim, David, Tina and Barb. Yes, my parents were pretty busy during those 10 years.   My father, Arnold, was in the Air Force for 20 years, and we moved around a lot when I was growing up. You could say I was a military brat. We lived in Nebraska, Arizona, Michigan, Colorado, Nevada and Oklahoma. Most of my fondest memories were when we were stationed in Oklahoma, from 1967 to 1976. I had the most wonderful friends and went to schools that were diverse, which taught me a lot about respecting all races.

My dad passed away in 1996, from a massive heart attack. He was only 59.   I miss him and think of him daily. My mom lives in an assisted living facility here in Colorado. Her memory is great, despite many ailments that come with aging. She has had both knees replaced, and suffers from neuropathy and arthritis. My parents must have done something right, because all of their children are wonderful, stable adults with loving partners.

Chapter 2

The Early Years

Melody and I met in March of 2000, I was 39 years old and she was 47. I was working for an electronics company and had a contract labor business at home. Melody was working at an insurance company as a Medicare customer service representative. She had her master's degree in communication, although she wasn't working in that field.

Our first few years together were very pleasant. We both enjoyed traveling and vacationed in Canada, as well as many trips to northern and southern California. We participated in many activities such as camping, dancing, entertaining, sporting events and concerts.

I was in the process of buying a new condo in Lakewood, Colorado in early 2002, when Melody was laid off. We had been dating for over two years, and decided it was the right time to take our relationship to the next level, and move in together. The transition was smooth, and we settled into our new life together.

Melody suffered from an eye condition called iritis, which is an inflammation of the eye. It can cause vision loss and/or glaucoma. She was having trouble driving and didn't feel comfortable driving long distances, so she looked for employment that was close to our condo. Melody found a job as a Medicare representative which was only a couple of miles from our place. She was working there for about a year. The company required their employees to take a written test annually for updated Medicare procedures. Melody had taken this test before with her previous employer and was optimistic that she would do fine. She flunked the test and was devastated. We assumed it was her iritis acting up. The company accommodated her by installing a larger monitor and better lighting. On her second attempt, she failed the test again, and was let go two weeks later. She was very depressed and I felt terrible for her. A few days after she was let go, a co-worker of hers called me and said that Melody had been forgetting things, and was not able to hold a conversation with her clients on the phone. I didn't really think much about it at the time, and didn't tell Melody about this.

Melody would have her eyes checked three times per year, so I made an appointment with her optometrist to see if her iritis was getting worse. He told us that her eyes were pretty inflamed but not to the point that it would be causing any major problems. When we got home, we talked about what she should do next. She wasn't feeling confident about driving anymore, so I suggested she take some time off to compose herself and apply to businesses in the neighborhood that she could walk to.

Looking back, there were many clues that other things were going on. There were minor memory lapses during our first few years together, which I attributed to her iritis and early menopause, which she was very much going through. I used to tease her about all her menopause symptoms, and she would tell me to just wait. Today, I know exactly what she was talking about, and I'm sure most menopausal women can relate!

There was one episode I recall when we were spending Christmas Eve, 2002, at my sister's place in Colorado Springs. My mother called me a few days later and said that Melody was having problems counting the dice when we were all playing Yahtzee. We had all been drinking a bit that night, and I assumed it was because of that.

In the meantime, I was going through my own health problems. I was having severe arthritis pain in my hips, heart palpitations and a lot of sleeplessness. I ended up in the emergency room one day when I became very dizzy at a restaurant in Colorado Springs. My sister and mother took me to the E.R. They did an EKG and found an abnormality in my heart. I followed up with my primary care physician and we went over my symptoms. After a few blood tests, I was diagnosed with a condition called hemochromatosis. The doctor explained that this condition causes your body to absorb too much iron. The iron is stored in your joints and organs, especially your heart, liver and pancreas. I was 43 years old, and had all of the symptoms, such as fatigue, joint pain and weakness. Also, x-rays showed that I was bone to bone on both of my hips.

Since I had this disease, chances are a parent or sibling also had it. My mom and siblings were all tested. They all tested negative except my brother David who was diagnosed. Since my father died of a massive heart attack at the age of 59, it is very probable he had this disease as well. In the 1990's, hemochromatosis wasn't a very well-known disease. I started having regular phlebotomies to reduce some of the iron in my bloodstream and was prescribed anti-inflammatory pain pills. I was in a significant amount of pain, but my main focus was on Melody.

Melody eventually walked to a few businesses in our neighborhood to fill out applications. One day when I got home from work, she was sitting on the couch, acting very disoriented and scared. She said she got lost and couldn't find her way home. Melody ended up at our beauty salon across the street from where we lived. Our beautician Kathy calmed her down and brought her home.

Since no one would hire her, in October of 2004, Melody filed for disability. She thought her eyes were getting worse and was feeling a lot of anxiety. It took over seven months to hear back from the state, and in May of 2005 we received a letter from the state denying her claim. The next month, I called a disability attorney so he could help us re-file her claim. We sat down with him to go over Melody's medical condition and the paperwork needed to file. Melody couldn't remember anything the attorney asked her about the places she worked and her eye problems. After the meeting, we were walking out of his office and he pulled me aside. He said that there was much more going on besides her eye condition. He told me to look down at Melody's feet. I approached her, looked down, and noticed she had her shoes on the wrong feet. It was at that moment that our lives changed forever.

Chapter 3

The Diagnosis

The attorney wanted Melody to see a neuropsychologist to get evaluated. I called and talked to one in Lakewood. He explained that he would do an evaluation which would include pencil and paper tests. The tests would assess a number of areas including intelligence, functions such as planning, memory, language, perception, motivation, mood and personality styles. The tests usually take between 3 and 6 hours. I explained all of this to Melody and she was fine with it. We both wanted answers, good or bad.

We arrived at the neuropsychologist's building and he greeted us. We proceeded to his office and he asked us to come in and sit down. He sat down on the chair by his desk, and Melody walked over to him and sat on his lap. I was so embarrassed, but he was very professional. He took her by the hand and led her to a chair a few feet away. Melody didn't comprehend what she had done and we never spoke about it. We went over symptoms, family history and feelings that Melody was having. She told him that she had not been feeling like herself and he suggested we proceed with the tests. He asked me to leave and check back in about three hours. I didn't have a good feeling about things. With the recent shoe incident and Melody sitting on his lap, I knew something serious was going on.

About two hours later I received a call from the receptionist to come back and pick up Melody. When I got there, she was sitting with the receptionist, having a cup of coffee. The doctor asked to talk to me in private. He told me that he stopped the tests because Melody was getting really frustrated and not comprehending anything. He said he would call back in the next few days with the results.

I could tell that Melody was upset so I suggested we drive up to Blackhawk for a few hours. That put a smile on her face. We both enjoyed occasional gambling and it was a good escape for us. We had a wonderful time and ended up getting a room for the night.

It was about three days later that I received a call from the doctor. He wanted me to take a look at the results. The first thing out of his mouth was that Melody was having very serious memory problems, most likely caused by dementia. He showed me a few of the tests, one in particular. It was called a clock draw test, where the person was supposed to draw a clock that read 3:00. Melody drew a circle. One hand was drawn outside of the circle, and the other hand was a straight line drawn across the inside of the circle. He said this test was a very useful screening tool that detected dementia or Alzheimer's. I found this very disturbing, and I knew right at that moment that Melody had dementia. He was very concerned and suggested that she get a CT scan immediately.

Melody had the CT scan, and was diagnosed with early onset dementia in 2006. She was 53 years old. We sat down to talk about how we would pursue this challenging diagnosis. She told me that it would be all right if I left her. She said that she knew what I was going to go through because she experienced the progression with her mother. I responded "Where would I go?" and told her that we needed each other. We held each other and cried for most of the evening.

Chapter 4

Daily Chores

2006 and part of 2007 were good for Melody. Her primary physician prescribed Melody a medication called memantine, which is used to treat moderate to severe dementia of the Alzheimer's type. He told us that the medication often gives some degree of improvement in memory or aspects of cognitive problems. One of the first things I did was take the car keys away and she was fine with that. As I mentioned before, Melody wasn't comfortable with driving so I didn't even need to convince her that it was time to give this up.

My employer let me switch to four days a week, 10-hour days. This allowed me to have more days with Melody at home. I worked for a small company and most of them didn't know what I was dealing with. I did confide in one co-worker who was very supportive. It was very therapeutic to be able to talk to someone on the bad days. I gave Melody chores to do during the day while I was at work. We had three cats: Scully, Ripley and Izzadora. One of her chores was to keep their food bowls filled. The dry food was tiny pebbles, so she called them "hardballs." She also cleaned the cat hair off of the furniture. From the time I left for work until I got home, Melody would clean cat hair from the furniture and every corner of the house. You would never know we had three cats! I would always compliment her about this and she would smile from ear to ear.

I read how important it is to help your loved one with memory games and also to monitor how the disease is progressing, so we would practice counting from 0 to 50, and I would have her recite the months of the year. I tested her almost every night. As those few years went by and Melody's condition progressed, she could sometimes make it to 50, and remembered all the months, but not in order.

One change I noticed in Melody was that she would repeat herself constantly. This was one area where I grew very impatient and agitated. There were times that I was so tired and would tell her to please stop and raised my voice. She would stop for a while and then start right back up again. She also would pace back and forth throughout the condo. She could not sit still, but when it came time for bed she was usually exhausted and slept most of the night. My work schedule was 5:00 a.m. to 3:00 p.m., Monday through Thursday. We would get up at 4:00 a.m., and I would get her breakfast, which consisted of a granola bar, yogurt and of course coffee, her favorite thing on the planet! I would make her lunch the night before, which was a sandwich and chips. By this time, she was not safe using the stove because a few times she had left the burners on. I had to remove the knobs and hide them so she wouldn't try to cook. I would call her a few times during the day while I was working to see how she was doing. Most days were good but sometimes she would accidentally hang up on me, I assumed, or maybe she just didn't want to talk anymore!

Melody only weighed around 100 pounds, but she loved to eat! She could eat anything, anytime and not gain a pound. We had a favorite steak house in Lakewood so every other Friday we would have lunch there. She loved the chicken and rice, and would always order a beer. The doctor told us to limit her alcohol intake, but I didn't want to take away everything she loved, and she did love her beer! The waitresses knew us very well and never had to ask Melody what she wanted. They all knew she had dementia and were awesome with her. Melody also loved wintergreen lifesavers. I kept a candy dish full of them on the coffee table so she could have a few while doing her chores daily. A few turned into *A LOT*. The candy dish would be empty by the time I returned home from work each day. I think she was also stashing them. I found lifesavers under her pillow, in her pant pockets, and in her sock drawer. I was thinking that the sugar was causing her anxiety and stress so I started limiting her to ten lifesavers a day. MELODY WAS NOT HAPPY!!!!

There was one incident that I will never forget, which was just fascinating. I called her one afternoon and asked her how she was doing. She told me that she had arranged all of the trash and put everything in order. I had no idea what I would find when I got home. When I entered the door, she greeted me with so much excitement about her accomplishment for the day. I walked into the kitchen and couldn't believe what I saw. She had taken all of the trash like paper, kleenex, coffee filters, etc. and put them in separate piles. It was quite a mess but by God she had each product arranged in the correct pile. I complimented her and she was so very proud of herself. It is amazing to me how the brain works. She could barely count to 50 yet she could be so meticulous in arranging everything in order.

Our cat Ripley was having kidney problems and we had to put her on dialysis twice a week for a few months. I called Melody one afternoon and she was frantic. She said Ripley wasn't moving and had been making strange noises all morning. I rushed home and took Ripley to the vet. Her kidneys had failed so we had to make that tough decision, and on May 8th, 2006 we had Ripley euthanized. Melody took this very hard. She felt that if she had been able to drive, she could have taken Ripley to the vet sooner and saved her life. The vet insisted that it wouldn't have mattered, but Melody was inconsolable for a very long time.

Chapter 5

Mary's Surgery

There were days when you would never know Melody had dementia, and days where you could see the disease so clearly. We had some great friends we hung out with regularly, but as her dementia progressed, many of them disappeared. They told me that they couldn't handle watching her deteriorate. I could truly understand. Two friends that were there for the duration were Beth and Joyce. They were our neighbors in the condo where we lived. Beth is an occupational therapist who works everyday with dementia and Alzheimer's patients. She started noticing changes in Melody before I did, but she couldn't convince me that it was more than her iritis.

There were a few times that Joyce would stay overnight with Melody while I went to visit my family in Colorado Springs. It was hard for Melody to make the trip without getting confused and agitated, and she didn't like to leave our cats. She enjoyed having Joyce stay with her. I think it was because of Joyce's calming voice.

Melody was doing pretty good, so in August of 2007 I decided to have my right hip replaced. The pain had become excruciating and I could barely function. Melody understood and said she would be fine for the three days that I would be hospitalized. I made arrangements for Beth to come up before and after work to check on Melody and spend time with her.

I talked to Melody quite often during my stay in the hospital and she seemed to be doing fine. My brother Tim picked me up from the hospital and brought me home. When we walked in the condo, Melody went ballistic. She wanted to know why I left her and said that she hadn't slept for days.   Tim and I sat her down and reminded her that I was in the hospital. She didn't remember anything about my surgery. After a few hours I was able to calm her down.

I took five weeks off of work. Beth would come in the evenings to help us both out. She was awesome. My hip healed very well. I knew that eventually I would need to get my left one replaced as well.

Chapter 6

Beth and Joyce's Stories

Beth and Joyce would like to share some funny and troubling stories about their time with Melody.

BETH

I have been working as an occupational therapist in geriatrics since 1994. In that time I have worked with many people who have had dementia. Although a variety of things can cause dementia, the outcome is often similar. A person is robbed of his or her ability to learn new things, to remember and to problem solve. They are progressively robbed of their ability to complete daily tasks.

I saw Melody's world get smaller and smaller as her dementia progressed. She had problems doing her job and was let go. She then gave up driving and her independent access to the community. Gradually she didn't want to leave our condominium community. I remember her taking on the domestic chores at home. It was important for her to be an equally providing partner. As her downstairs neighbor, I watched her get the mail, take out the trash and care for the cats.

Looking back, I remember Mary telling me that Mel was having some problems that they thought might be related to menopause and her eye condition. I remember several incidences that led me to believe it was more than that.

The first one happened when I was on my way to the mailbox and she was standing near the mailroom looking around. I asked her where she was headed and she said she wanted to go home. I asked her if she knew which way to go and she responded "NO." I helped her get back to her place.

The second incident happened when Mel was in my condo, helping me care for my sick kitten Tess. I needed someone to hold her while I put medicine in her mouth. Melody picked up Tess and readied her for me. She was holding Tess upside down. Mel had no idea she was holding Tess that way and she needed help turning her in the right position. When it was time for her to leave, she couldn't find the front door of my 780-square-foot condo. I knew that night that Mel had more going on than vision problems.

The final incident that solidified my suspicions was one morning when I was getting ready for work. I was blow-drying my hair and noticed water running down my wall. I knew Melody was upstairs alone since Mary left very early for work every morning. I called upstairs and asked her if everything was all right. She told me that her socks were wet. I immediately went up to find the kitchen sink faucet turned on and water was spilling onto the counter and overflowing onto the floor. There was at least an inch of water covering the kitchen floor. Mel didn't comprehend why her socks were wet or where the water was coming from. I knew then that she probably had some kind of dementia.

Soon Mel was diagnosed with dementia and needed more and more help. Mary hired me to go up every morning and help Mel get ready for the day. I remember one day I went up and she had had a bowel movement on the living room floor. I quietly cleaned it up and then casually helped her into the bathroom to get cleaned up. I always tried to preserve her dignity by acting like nothing was amiss, and ask for her permission to help her with things.

It's peculiar what dementia takes and what it leaves behind. One thing that struck me was when I would help Mel wash her hands. She needed help to find the sink, turn the water on and get the soap on her hands. The one thing she did remember was the healthiest way to wash hands. She would scrub the front and back of her hands, as well as weave her fingers to get in between them. She would then scrub her finger tips against the palm of her hands. She rivaled a surgeon scrubbing in for surgery! I always complimented her, and she would say; "That's the way to get the *ick* off." Looking at her hands while she washed made me think about how her hands still connected to her brain that was once whole, wise and knowing.

What amazed me about Mel, as compared to some other people with dementia, was that she was able to discuss her condition. She would tell me that she had dementia and that her mother probably had it too. I would ask her how she felt knowing that she had dementia. She would always say that " It is what it is and there is nothing I can do about it so I am not going to get upset." She indicated that she would just face it head on. I had so much respect for her. The one gift that came with Mel's disease is that she really had no insight in to how much help she needed and how debilitated she had become. She would often say "I think I am doing pretty well." I would always agree with her. One task that made her feel useful and productive was when she would take the lint brush and rub it around on the furniture. She felt helpful in cleaning up the cat hair. No matter how grumpy I was in the morning Mel could always cheer me up. She was afraid that strangers would come in and when she heard the door open she would yell "Who is it?" As soon as she heard my voice or saw my face she would smile and get excited.

JOYCE

In addition to her outside job, Mary had a home business and I began helping her out as well as spending the day with Mel while Mary was at work. She cracked me up one day when I got there. She said that BAD Mary was there last night and boy was she mad! It took me a minute to figure out what she was talking about, but I thought it was so funny how she described it. She said that GOOD Mary was here this morning but not last night. I said something like "We can't all have good days all the time." She said she didn't know about that, but she was glad when bad Mary left!

I have fond memories of the times we hung out together. She would walk around and clean the furniture with her lint brush. She loved giving the cats their "hardball" food and making sure the bowls were filled. She loved drinking coffee. When she got agitated you could always fix her a cup of coffee and it would distract her for a while. When we learned that she shouldn't drink a lot of coffee, my first thought was wondering what we would do now to help calm her down.

A few times when I was working in Mary's work room Mel would come in and say people were trying to get in through the windows and doors. I would make sure that everything was locked and assured her that we were safe. I told her that if anyone came in that we would kick them and take them out to the trash. We would practice how we would kick them. I assured her that we were strong women and that we could take on anyone that tried to mess with us, except bad Mary!

One night I spent the night with Mel, when Mary went to visit her family. Mary told me that when it was time to go to bed, just lay down with her until she falls asleep. We were in there only a few minutes when she told me that I wasn't Mary and she got out of bed. There was no way she was going to lay there with me. Eventually she did fall asleep on the couch, but I still laugh when I think about that! We tried to keep the routine but she knew I was not supposed to be there next to her.

Chapter 7

Changes in Melody

I always assumed dementia and Alzheimer's disease were the same. That is not the case. Dementia isn't a disease in itself. It is a group of symptoms which affect mental tasks like memory and reasoning. Dementia can be caused by a variety of conditions, the most common of which is Alzheimer's. Beth explained to me that there are five stages of progression in dementia. The first stage is no noticeable impairment. Stage two is minor memory inconsistencies. Stage three is when the person becomes disoriented and suffers from short-term memory loss that disrupts aspects of the day. The fourth stage is when the person can't care for most of their daily needs and must be accompanied. The final stage is when the person can't function at all without constant assistance, and has extreme memory loss.

Melody was now showing symptoms of stage three. I will never forget one night when we were sitting on the couch watching a movie. Out of the blue, she said, "Oh, there's Handsome." I thought she was talking about someone in the movie. She was trying to get our cat Scully to jump up on the couch next to her. I was dumbfounded and told her that she was talking to Scully, and she insisted his name was Handsome. From then on, Scully was Handsome.

I was beginning to notice a lot of changes in Melody that were not particularly common with dementia. The first incident that concerned me was one morning when we woke up. Melody was having trouble getting out of bed. Her legs didn't want to work. I went around the bed to get her in an upright position, and I noticed that her upper body and head were leaning to the right. I thought she might have a backache. This continued off and on during the duration of her battle.

The next incident was when I returned home from work one day, and found Melody pacing around in the kitchen. She was completely naked with her feces all over her. She told me that she had an accident in the living room. She had tried to clean it up but made more of a mess. I don't even think she realized that she was covered in her own feces. I immediately took her to the shower and cleaned her up.

The third incident was one day when I came home from work and saw a business card on the kitchen table. The card contained the name and number of a Lakewood police officer. I asked Melody where it came from. She said the police came over looking for the man that was in the condo. I called the officer. He informed me that someone in the neighborhood had called 911 to say that Melody was standing by the sliding glass door screaming that someone was trying to get her. The officer arrived and tried to calm her down. He searched the condo and assured her that there was no one there. I explained to him that she had dementia and he was very sympathetic. He did tell me that she shouldn't be left alone during the day, and he was concerned for her safety.

The final few incidences started one evening when we were getting ready for bed. Melody walked into the bathroom to brush her teeth. All of a sudden she started screaming that the man was back and was staring at her. I ran into the bathroom. She was pointing at the mirror, yelling "There he is!" She was looking at her own reflection, thinking it was the man who had been following her. It took me a long time to calm her down and explain that she was looking at herself. She couldn't comprehend this. I took a white plastic bag and covered the mirror. This helped for a few days, until one evening when the phone rang. Melody stood up to answer it, and when she picked up the receiver, she looked up at the wall. "There he is!!!" she screamed, and dropped the phone. She was hysterical, pointing to the wall, which had a picture in a glass frame. Again she saw a reflection of herself, this time in the glass, thinking it was the man. As a precaution I removed all of the pictures in our condo, regardless of whether they were in a glass frame.

Chapter 8

Total Longterm Care Center

I was extremely emotionally drained and exhausted. There was no way I could leave Melody home alone while I was at work any longer. Reality hit me at this time knowing Melody wasn't going to get better. In the past, Melody and I had discussed that we both wanted to be cremated, so I registered us with a local cremation facility. I completed Melody's living will, and became her medical and financial power of attorney.

I knew there were many resources for help out there. The first person I thought of for advice was Beth. We both sat down and talked about the options and resources. Beth suggested Melody start going to Total Longterm Care Center of Lakewood where she worked. This would be an excellent facility because Beth could drop in and visit Melody during the day. Melody loved Beth and felt safe around her.

Melody started going to the center in mid-2008. They were awesome. Melody was assigned a new primary doctor and a counselor for both of us. She went there Monday through Thursday, 8am to 3pm. The bus picked her up and brought her home. I hired Beth to come up in the mornings to get her ready. I would be home when Melody got home in the afternoon. It took a few weeks for her to adjust, sometimes resisting but in general she enjoyed the time with other adults and the attention she got from the staff. Having Beth around helped a lot. Here is an experience Beth had with Melody.

One morning I went upstairs to help Mel get ready for the care center before I went to work. She was on her hands and knees and couldn't tell me why. It didn't seem as though she had fallen but rather had purposely gotten down on the floor. I told her I was going to help her get up and initially she agreed. When I tried to help her stand up she went into a full-blown panic attack and starting screaming and fighting me. I let go and she got back on her hands and knees. I couldn't figure out what was wrong. I tried a few more times to get her up and again she became terrified and kept screaming. I called the center and told them the circumstances. The doctor wanted to see her. A co-worker, Patty who is also an occupational therapist agreed to come over and help. We tried several times to lift Mel off of the floor but terror overtook her every time. Patty and I had an idea. Thinking Mel was having something called gravitational insecurity we thought sandwiching her between us would make her feel more secure as we helped her stand. We knelt down and put Mel between us. Patty's back was to Mel and we asked her to hold onto Patty's shoulders. I was in the back ready with my hands on

Mel's waist to help lift her. We decided to stand really close like an Oreo cookie and all stand up together. As we started to stand, Mel again became terrified and began screaming. Patty and I kept lifting. Mel then took her hands off Patty's shoulders and grabbed her around the chest. In doing that she accidently grabbed a hold of Patty's breast. For one brief funny moment, Mel stopped and said, "Oh, this is nice." The three of us had a good laugh. We ended up calling 911 and the firefighters got her up. Beth then drove Melody to the center to see the doctor.

Since Melody was attending the center daily, I decided to have my right hip replaced. This would be the perfect opportunity because I could recover and not worry about her during the day. I made arrangements with Melody's niece Angie to fly out from Arizona and stay with Melody for the three days that I would be hospitalized. Angie arrived the day before my surgery, and was so surprised how much Melody had deteriorated in the last few years since they had last seen each other. It was really hard for Angie to see her aunt in this condition and she was ready to leave after the second day. This was the last time they saw each other.

Melody was doing great at the center for over a year but started having problems walking up and down the stairs in our third story condo. She was also getting very impatient getting to the bus. It would take 45 minutes for the bus driver to get her down the stairs. She would get frantic thinking she was going to fall. The bus accommodated up to seven clients, most of them suffering from dementia or Alzheimer's. The driver would make stops to pick up other clients after picking up Melody. She would get very impatient and agitated sitting on the bus for long periods of time. Other clients would as well but Melody seemed to be the worst. She would yell and try to get out of her seat.

The staff decided to have the driver pick up Melody last in the mornings and I would pick her up after work. This helped tremendously for a while but then Melody started acting out when she was at the center. When someone tried to socialize with her, she would get in their face and yell. She used profanity and also began kicking if anyone got too close to her.

In late August of 2009, I received a call from the care center. The staff wanted to have a consultation with me. I knew right away what the outcome was going to be. The staff made a decision that Melody really needed to be placed in assisted living. Her dementia was really progressing. They asked my thoughts about it. I remember feeling angry thinking they didn't want to deal with Melody anymore and that they didn't care. I felt as though we all failed her. I was told that it is very common for caregivers to react in this way. I had known this day would come but didn't want to accept the fact that Melody wasn't going to be around much longer.

Placing Melody in assisted living was the hardest decision I have ever had to make in my life. At age 49, I had to place my partner, age 56, in assisted living. The care center staff located a house that was converted into an assisted living facility, Ashley Manor, which accommodated up to 12 clients. The majority of them had some form of dementia. The facility would be a very short distance from our condo. They wanted to move her in the next few weeks. I had no idea how I was going to approach Melody with this.

Chapter 9

Assisted Living

I thought the easiest way to approach this was to ask Melody for a favor. I told her that I really needed her to stay at an assisted living facility during the week because I was working a lot and wouldn't get home from work until later in the evenings. I didn't want to use the word "move" thinking that would really upset her. I promised that she could come home every weekend to care for the cats and help me around the condo. I couldn't believe her reaction. She was so excited to help, thinking that if she didn't contribute, then we would all be separated.

The move was harder for me than Melody. I don't think she comprehended what was going on. I was a mess. I tried not to get emotional around her, so at times I would go into a different room and have a good cry.

Melody moved into the assisted living facility in September of 2009. I spent most of the morning getting her settled in. She didn't like her new room and I tried to reassure her that she would come home in a few days. The staff suggested that I leave that afternoon. They thought Melody would settle down if I wasn't around.

The next morning I received a call saying Melody intentionally threw herself to the floor when the aide was taking her to the bathroom. She split open the bridge of her nose and had a pretty nasty bump on her forehead. They were keeping an eye on her to make sure she had not suffered a concussion.

The staff was also noticing the shuffled walk, rigid muscle tremors, and hallucinations. They suspected that there were issues going on in addition to dementia. They recommended Melody see her primary doctor. After a physical and discussing her symptoms with me, the doctor came to the conclusion that Melody most likely had Lewy Bodies Dementia. He told me that LBD is the second most common type of progressive dementia after Alzheimer's disease. He said that LBD is hard to diagnose. To be diagnosed with LBD you must have experienced a progressive decline in your ability to think as well as two of the following:

1: Fluctuating alertness and thinking (cognitive) function.

2: Repeated visual hallucinations.

3: Parkinson's symptoms (rigid muscles, slowed movement and tremors).

Melody had all of these symptoms.

I went to visit Melody the following afternoon after work. She believed Handsome was falling apart and wanted him to stay with her. The facility didn't allow pets, but I had promised her that Handsome could stay with her. I went to a toy store and purchased a stuffed cat that actually moved and meowed. I brought it into Melody's room hoping she would think it was Handsome. She looked at it, rolled her eyes and tossed it to the side. Beth had just arrived and asked Melody how Handsome was. We didn't think Melody knew it was a *fake cat,* but she knew it wasn't *her cat.* She informed us that "This cat needs a good brushing!" We all laughed and agreed.

The staff loved Melody and she loved them too, especially Tina and Nancy. They always made sure Melody had her coffee which was now decaf. I think they gave her a little bit more attention than anyone else. I would visit Melody almost every day after work. I kept my promise and brought Melody home on the weekends. Melody's good friend, Tammy, moved from Michigan to Denver about the same time Melody was placed in assisted living. She visited Melody often and noticed the decline from the last time she saw her in 2007. Tammy remembers one visit:

My sister Tracy and I were sitting with Melody on the balcony of the condo and she asked us for a cigarette. I gave her one. We were laughing and talking about the neighbors when Melody kept looking towards the entry door. It was like she was trying to hide something from someone inside. She smiled, giggled and said she was looking for Mary because she was not supposed to be smoking. Melody would also joke about her memory loss and yet you could see it was painful for her. She was well aware of her dementia at such an early age. She was a funny, caring, and sarcastic friend to all of us. She taught me how not to take life so seriously and always laugh, even when you felt like crying.

In October of 2009, my brother Tim called and asked if I would like to fly out to California the following June with him and his partner. He thought this would be a much needed getaway. I really could use a few days to relax and rejuvenate so we booked the flight. Melody's birthday, October 31st was awesome. I remember how happy she was. She ate lots of cake which surprised me since she didn't have a sweet tooth. She socialized and danced the day away. Thanksgiving and Christmas were exciting too. The staff bought all the clients Christmas pajamas and had one heck of a party.

In late January 2010, Melody was now using a wheel chair because her legs didn't want to work. It was hectic to get her up and down the stairs especially when none of the neighbors were around to help me. She started throwing tantrums when it was time to leave on Sundays. The staff insisted that I stop bringing her home. I knew this was the right decision. She was no longer socializing with anybody at Ashley Manor and would always yell out my name. She always wanted to talk to me. The staff would call me so Melody could hear my voice. This calmed her down but there were times I wasn't available to talk. One of the aides and I came up with an idea. We would record my voice on tape and when they couldn't reach me they would play the tape. My voice would tell her that she needed to calm down, get some rest so we could hang out together later. I would ramble on as if we were having a conversation. We didn't know if she comprehended what was going on but by gosh this worked.

In early April, Melody started declining rapidly. She was now confined to one area of the living room during the day. She would constantly rock in the recliner staring into space or yelling at the other clients if they got too close to her. She had lost all control of her bladder and bowels. One evening Melody had a complete breakdown. She was trying to get out of her wheelchair and started kicking at anything and anyone. The doctor suggested Melody go to a rehabilitation center to get evaluated and have her medications adjusted. I thought this was an awful suggestion but didn't have much of a choice. They said she had to either go to a rehab center for two weeks or be admitted into a nursing home.

The rehab center was located in Brighton, Colorado. They had very strict visiting hours: six hours daily from 8 to 11 am, and 2 to 5 pm. It was hard for me to visit during the week. Tammy's work schedule was very flexible so she would visit Melody almost every other morning and I would visit her every other afternoon. I went to see her the Saturday before her release and couldn't believe how much she had deteriorated . She was disoriented, had no idea who I was, couldn't sit up, and refused to eat. I thought it was the medication changes, but her nurse told me Melody was probably in her last stages of life, maybe 2 to 3 months.

At this point Ashley Manor thought the best care Melody would receive would be in hospice. Melody was admitted to hospice at Bethany Nursing Home in late April, 2010.

Chapter 10

Hospice

Melody was now only eating pureed food and had no idea who I was or where she was. She slept most of the time or would sit up in her wheelchair and mumble words. I would visit every evening and help feed her.

My trip to California was coming up. I was **really** struggling with deciding if I should go or cancel the trip. All my friends insisted I go. Hospice told me Melody would be fine and thought I really needed to get away. Tammy promised she would visit Melody each day and if there were any changes she would call me. I felt guilty leaving but knew Melody was in good hands. I flew out on June 1st. During my visit, I called hospice and Tammy daily.

I returned home late Sunday night, June 6th and was looking forward to visiting Melody. I had just arrived at work Monday morning when my cell phone rang. It was hospice, saying that Melody had taken a turn for the worse and told me to get there as soon as possible. I left work right away and stopped by the nurse's station as soon as I arrived. The nurse told me Melody had a day or two left. I had prepared myself for this day. I was sad but also relieved that Melody wouldn't be suffering much longer.

Melody was unresponsive, her breathing was labored and her feet and legs were reddish purple. Hospice was giving her morphine to keep her as comfortable as possible. The nurse explained to me what Melody was experiencing. Physically her body was beginning the final process of shutting down, which will end when all physical systems cease to function. These changes are a normal natural way in which the body prepares itself to stop. The reddish purple streaks were caused by lack of blood circulation, which is called mottling.

Melody was also going through the emotional, spiritual-mental process. The hospice nurse explained that the spirit begins the final process of release from the body. Melody very likely was confronting and resolving issues from her past. She was moaning a little bit which the nurse said is common during the spiritual process.

This process continued for most of the week. I didn't leave Melody's side except to go home to shower and get a few hours of sleep. Beth and Tammy spent a lot of time with Melody too. For some reason, I sensed there was something keeping Melody from letting go. I held her hand and told her I would be all right if she let go. Thursday morning Beth came to visit before she went to work. She was also wondering why Melody was still holding on. She thought it would be a great idea to run home and get Handsome's blanket he slept on. When she got back we placed the blanket on Melody's chest, thinking this might be what she needed. Friday morning I took some of Handsome's fur from the blanket, placed it up against her nose and then placed the fur in her hand. I kept telling Melody that Handsome and I would take care of each other and she need not worry.

Melody lost her battle a few hours later at 12:31 pm, Friday June 11th, 2010. She was 57 years old.

WHEN MELODY TOOK HER LAST BREATH, I TOOK MY FIRST BREATH IN A VERY LONG TIME.

.

Epilogue

I think quite often of Melody and hope that she and her sister Dawn are holding hands and having their time together now.

I have often wondered which was harder for me, losing my father so suddenly or watching Melody suffer for so many years. I never was able to say goodbye to my father but did get to say goodbye to Melody. Both experiences were extremely tough and I have come to the conclusion that the grieving process is extremely difficult regardless of the circumstances.

I have met some wonderful friends since Melody's passing. I still have a friendship with Beth, Joyce and Tammy. They are my angels. Their support meant the world to me.

During my years of caring for Melody, I lost my identity. My whole life was focused on the role of caregiver. After Melody went into assisted living, I was lost because my whole world had been caring for her, so I didn't know what to do with myself. I felt helpless and alone. My grieving process began at this time. I started working out regularly which helped me clear my mind and focus on myself again.

One of my new friends, Beverly and I went on a cruise to Cozumel and the Cayman Islands in April of 2011. I always wanted to swim with the dolphins and got that opportunity in Cozumel. Wow, what an experience swimming and socializing with these amazing mammals. Melody always knew I wanted to do this and I'm sure she was looking down smiling.

Handsome passed away on September 13th, 2011 a little over a year after Melody passed. He was 17 years old.

In March of 2012, I met the most wonderful woman, Stacie. She works with special needs children in the school system, and has a 14-year-old daughter, Brianna. I have been blessed with these two amazing people in my life.

Writing this book has brought the closure I needed, along with the support and love from my family and friends.

About the Author

Mary Kristofek was born in Tucson, Arizona in 1960. She has lived in Colorado for the last 40 years and calls Colorado home.

She has worked in the electronics Industry for over 35 years.

Mary loves to vacation, especially in California. She enjoys the outdoors, dining out, and time with family and friends.

She found tremendous healing journaling about her time caring for Melody. Stacie encouraged Mary to share her story which offers a portrait of life as a caregiver for someone with dementia. This is Mary's first book.

.